MW00831701

Thank God I Got Cancer…

I'm Not a Hypochondriac Anymore!

ANGELINA ASSANTI

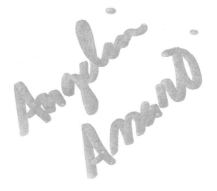

This book was written to make light of a serious subject. The author is not qualified to give advice on dating, never mind anything as serious as cancer. Please seek medical attention for diagnosis or treatment. The statements made by the author do not reflect those of the publishing company.

Cover photo by Jadlynn Scott

ISBN-13: 978-0692568255

ACKNOWLEDGMENTS

Jacobs Writing Consultants,
' the official editing service for
The City of Palms Publishing Company.

Copy Editor
Laurence Ruble

DEDICATION

This book is dedicated to my medical team, my fellow cancer survivors, cancer patients and their caretakers.

Please don't lose your sense of humor!

The Worst Year of My Life

We were only a month into 2015 and I already declared it the worst year of my life. In August of 2014, my husband and I were driving back from a fabulous weekend at the Waldorf-Astoria in Boca Raton when I got a phone call that would be the first bad news in a long line of terrible things to come. I have not put all of my hardships I faced at this time in my life, in this book. After all, I hardly know you!

My grandmother had a stroke and was in the ICU. They didn't know how bad she was. I told my mom we were on our way back home. My grandparents were not in great health but they were maintaining their independence. This would be really difficult for my grandfather. He was legally blind and his hearing was not that great, even with hearing aids. We offered to take him in so he didn't have to be alone. He refused.

As the weeks went by, I drove him to the hospital every day to check on my grandmother. The doctor told us they would have to release her to a nursing home because grandpa could not give her the kind of care she would need. She was in a nursing home for six weeks. While we were there we observed a ward down the hall from her room. It was the lockdown ward. That was where they put the people suffering from dementia and Alzheimer's disease. We were so glad she didn't have either of those. Those patients were loaded up with so much medicine they were like zombies. We all agreed no one should have to live like that. There must be nothing worse than being a prisoner in your own mind. As the months went by my grandmother recovered and went back to the apartment she shared with my grandfather.

December 2014

My cat, Samson, had a lump on his chest. I was not

concerned about it. He'd had a lipoma five years previously and we were told it was going to come back. A few weeks went by and I noticed it had gotten huge. It was time to take Samson to the vet. As soon as the vet touched him he told us a lump like that is always cancerous. I should have taken him right in. I really thought it was his lipoma coming back. He did not have any symptoms. I had noticed he was drinking a lot of water – a lot. But he was eating like a little pig, as he always did. So, I did not have any cause for concern. The doctor suggested surgery and sent his tumor away to a pathologist who would tell us exactly what it was. Okay, I will stop this story and tell you - *there's a reason why I'm telling you about my cat's cancer.* Weeks went by and the prognosis was good. I was thrilled because we rescued Samson eight years ago and he was an awesome cat.

Meanwhile, for my grandfather, the news would not be so good. My mom drove him and my grandmother to the hospital because he had chronic shoulder pain. Still a sharp guy, we were confident he would be out in a few hours. When my mom called me later that night, she told me he'd been admitted. I went to see him the next day and I think that was the last time he knew who I was.

They had a psychologist and neurologist visit him, and they told us he had dementia and would never be coming home. Grandpa had a tough life. He was one of eleven children and his mom put him and two of his siblings in an orphanage because she could not afford all of them. Grandpa was never one to show affection. Maybe that's where I get it from.

I know what you're thinking – I thought this was supposed to be a *funny* book. We are getting there. I need to give you background information first so you know my frame of mind when all this was going on. Don't worry, it gets funny when I'm diagnosed with cancer.

God, that is sad!

My mom researched the residential care facilities in the area and made an educated decision. One was sold to us as a rehab facility center. My grandfather was an active guy. We did not want him zombified like the patients at the rehab center where my grandmother went for her rehabilitation. We were told this too was a rehab facility and that he would be active and the staff would be interacting with him and giving him exercise. None of this was true. He wound up being confined to a wheelchair. Every time he would try and get up an alarm went off. They were not giving him exercise. They were not even providing decent meals. This facility was like punishment. It treated the patients with memory issues like prisoners. They kept them so drugged-up they were not even conscious most of the time.

Back to the cat

We got the pathology report back. By then the vet had already seen Samson for his post-op check-up and said it looked like Samson would be okay. They thought they removed all the cancer during his surgery. But, he had Fibrosarcoma, which is *always* terminal for cats and dogs. One month after the surgery the lump was back. This was absolutely devastating. The vet said we needed to put him down. There was nothing we could do. I would not hear of it. How did this happen? How do you prepare for devastating news when you were told there would be a different outcome?

I contacted a holistic doctor I know and tried a Native American recipe for healing. It looked like it was working for the first two weeks and then I woke up one morning and there was a huge mass that was red and his flesh was open. I called my husband and told him he had to take him in right away and put him down. Needless to say, it was devastating. I am literally dropping tears on my keyboard right now. Samson slept with me that last night, which he never did. I know he knew.

I was depressed for weeks. It was an emotional rollercoaster with a very bad ending. I will never forget how often I was filling up his water bowl during those months. He could not get satiated. And, I could not fix him. He was only eight when he died. Why couldn't it have happened to some stray cat that no one cared about? Why him? Sarcomas are very rare. Those account for only 1% of all cancers.

Three weeks after we put Samson down, we went to the shelter and adopted a calico cat. Her name was Rapunzel but she didn't answer to it and she was three years old. We talked about calling her 'Wildfire,' but that name got shortened to 'Wi-Fi' and for some reason, she answered to that right away.

April 2015

As the months went by we spent time with grandpa. He did not recognize us most of the time. In fact, we had to call the facility ahead of time and ask if he was awake. He was so doped up there was almost no point in going.

May 2015

Wow. I was really thirsty. No matter how much water I drank I could not quench my thirst. I thought about Samson and how thirsty he was towards the end. No, that's crazy. I live in Florida. It's hot. It's ninety-five degrees. I'm just dehydrated. Duh! I just need to stop drinking caffeinated beverages and I'll be fine. A couple weeks went by and I started thinking maybe I had diabetes. Dehydration is one of the signs. And there's a lot of diabetes in my family. Just a few years earlier, I had been diagnosed as a pre-diabetic. I'd better go to my doctor just to make sure I don't have the real deal this time. I'll feel much better when I go see my doctor, I thought.

I tried to get an appointment but it would be two weeks before I could get in. I'd better just see his physician's assistant. She could run some blood work, but more importantly, she could run a urinalysis and rule out diabetes. I was confident that she was going to tell me to just drink more water.

The day of the appointment comes. I'm drinking a lot of water to trick my kidneys into functioning properly (those suckers). I marvel at my genius. Although it's a twenty minute ride to the doctor, it's okay. I'm sure they'll give me the urinalysis right away so my bladder doesn't explode in the exam room. By the time I arrive I'm doing the pee-pee dance in the waiting room. Thank God they were running on time! The nurse walks me back to the exam room and asks me why I'm there. She then walks over to the table and is about to wrap the Velcro around my arm to take my blood pressure when I stop her. "Look, I don't mean to be rude, but I have to pee really badly! I know you're doing a urinalysis, so can I just pee in a cup now?" I asked, confident that she'd just hand the cup over.

"No, I need to get your blood pressure now. You can go after."

As I squirm, she slaps the cuff and a look of horror comes across her face. "Uh, I need to do that again. That can't be right," she says. Again, I squirm as I pray to God that I don't pee all over the examination table and she says, "I have to get the doctor."

"What's the matter?" I asked, seeing that she was panicked.

"You're blood pressure is 166 over 99. You're about to have a heart attack!" she squeals as she darts out the room.

Now my blood pressure was *really* climbing. "Oh God," I said, "I'm gonna have a heart attack *and* I still have to pee!" I yelled, "Can I go pee *now*?"

"Just pee in a cup in the bathroom," she yelled from around the corner.

I walked calmly to the bathroom to avoid a heart attack and peed in the cup. And let me tell you, my cup overfloweth. She was right. My heart was pounding. I could feel it throbbing all over. I looked at my chest and could see my shirt pulsating. I could not believe it. I was going to die in the doctor's office – maybe even on the *toilet*. I could picture the crowd at my memorial service, all eating grilled peanut butter and banana sandwiches, paying tribute to me and the King having both departed on the crapper.

Alas, I finished and washed my hands. The nurse was right outside the door to take my cup. No one with a defibrillator. That's good. Maybe I'm calming down. Maybe I won't have a heart attack. Yeah! I'll totally psyche myself out of my inevitable heart attack. I walked back to the exam room and an EKG machine awaited me. They wasted no time hooking me up to monitor my inevitable demise.

And the shocking results were in…I was not having a heart attack and my blood pressure returned to 120 over 80. So, what happened? Well, it just so happens that a friend of mine is a doctor. When I told him what had happened he was not impressed. Apparently, when you have to pee really badly your blood pressure goes way up. He said people sometimes pass out because of it. Oh, the bonus was my urinalysis came back normal. That did not stop the doctor's office from scheduling me to have further heart tests and checking my kidney function. After I spoke with my doctor friend I canceled everything my doctor's office had planned and decided I would find a different doctor. You know what is worse than a hypochondriac? A doctor's office who plays into it. Here's your takeaway, always pee before someone takes your blood pressure!

June 5

I had an abnormal mammogram. Today I have to go back for a follow-up exam. The technicians follow up my exam with an ultra-sound, which is the right thing to do. Not every mammography center does this. I have what is called, "Dense breast tissue." It's fatty. That makes it easier for tumors to hide. I think to myself, "Please, God. Don't let me have breast cancer." I shouldn't have been so specific. I did not have *breast* cancer.

June 10

I go to see my OB/GYN. We make small chit chat and then the exam begins. "I don't like what I'm seeing down here," he says.

"Sorry about that, I haven't been to the spa in a while," I said.

"No. You have a spot on your cervix. This looks like cancer."

That got my attention. "Cancer?" I asked. Ugh, I knew it was going to get me.

"Yes, a spot like this is always cancer. I will send this out for a biopsy and call you as soon as the result comes in. Just…be prepared," he said.

I did not have *one* symptom of cancer. Typical symptoms include the following: nausea, vomiting, fever, night sweats, diarrhea, loss of appetite, weight loss, swollen lymph nodes, fatigue, etc. I didn't have any idea. There were days that I wanted to take a nap, but most of the time I felt absolutely great. That was the most deceptive part. I still looked really healthy and felt great. The only clue I had was I was drinking water constantly like Samson. It felt like I was crawling in the desert seeking water.

June 11

I call the holistic doctor I know and she tells me to start taking spores made from an ancient mushroom that have been known to reverse cancer cells in some people.

June 13

It was grandpa's 90th birthday. We brought him a chocolate milkshake and had a little party for him. I thought he recognized me in a moment of lucidity when he looked excitedly and said, *"My GOD…"* He must have recognized me, I thought. Then, he continued, *"Did you get FAT!"*

I shrugged it off and said to my grandmother, "He must not know it's me."

She reassured me, "Oh, he knows it's you." Thanks, nana. I'm only a size eight. Give me a break.

July 3

The doctor calls and tells me to come into the office right

away. He also tells me to have someone drive me. That is never a good sign. I have never waited so long for test results to come in.

July 6

I'm telling my husband the whole way there that I have cancer and that I hope I'm going to be okay while he tries to convince me it's all in my head. If a doctor tells you to come to their office immediately and to bring a ride, it's not because he misses you. Obviously something is very wrong. My heart was pounding. My blood pressure was 140 over 90.

My doctor sat down and exhaled, "I'm sorry my dear, you have cancer." I could see the weight of this news on the doctor. I actually felt bad for him. I was glad I did not have a job where I had to tell people they had cancer.

"In your face! I told you I had cancer!" I said to my husband calmly.

"You were right," my husband said. He was more upset than I was. After all, the doctor had already told me the day of the exam. But, my husband thought I was being dramatic. The doctor raised an eyebrow at my response, as he watched my reaction and the exchange with my husband. Apparently other people cry when they are told they have cancer. I guess people don't like to be right as much as I do. As the doctor escorted me out of his office his nurse handed me an appointment card for the next day. They had already contacted an oncologist in Fort Myers and he assured me this cancer specialist was one of the best doctors he knew. He said, "Good luck," with a sympathetic smile and we were out the door.

The car ride home was pretty quiet. My husband was upset. We did not know how far along the cancer was. We did not know what the treatments were going to be. I was actually handling it better than my husband. I was receiving the inevitable bad news I always dreaded.

I was proud of my husband for refraining from dispensing his typical and solid medical advice of *"suck it up."* This was clearly beyond that point.

Guess what kind of cancer? A sarcoma, like my cat. Ooh, I'm finally part of the 1%. Yay me! My mom always told me I was special. Why did it have to be cancer?

By the way you're now the new leper to everyone you know. You may as well yell, "Unclean, unclean" at people when they start finding out you have cancer. Some people have yet to learn that cancer is not contagious. That is why I lick their face if they seem freaked out. Just kidding. That's gross. I don't know where their face has been. Just be prepared, people are ignorant. I hope this isn't news to you.

A Theme Song

I was driving out of my doctor's office when the song "Overcomer" by Mandisa came on the radio. That is my theme song for cancer. If you have been diagnosed, you need to pick a theme song, too. You need a fight song. Go ahead, pick "Eye of the Tiger," if it makes you feel better.

The song I picked actually had cancer survivors in its video. They are famous people who had cancer and are now cancer-free. But the lyrics are what got me. And you need to start thinking of yourself as an overcomer, too.

Let me just tell you now, I have never been a hugger.

I blame the great hugging tragedy of 1992. Here's where I've gone wrong of late. I made the mistake of telling people I'm not a hugger. There's even been a sport invented for it – "The Hugger Games." I don't know how many points you actually get when you land a hug on me. But it must be a lot. Because I get hugged…frequently. It's surprising too. Because when I see someone running towards me with open arms I turn into Keanu Reeves' character in the Matrix. You'd be surprised how far I can bend backwards to avoid a hug.

Guess what? When you have cancer some people want to hug you. They'd even ask. "Do you need a hug?" And I'd smile politely and say no thanks but usually it was too late. Before I knew it I was sighing while patting their back. This cancer thing is the beginning of a long hug-filled journey.

July 7

You have heard it said about war, there are no atheists in a foxhole. I submit to you that there are no atheists in oncologists' waiting rooms either. As I looked around the room I exchanged awkward smiles with the other patients. I had never been close to anyone who had cancer. I did not know what happened at an oncologist's office. I did not know what the treatments were like. I was totally ignorant. My husband went with me but had to leave during my appointment because he had a meeting and the appointment was so far behind schedule. He is partner in the firm he works at. He is always working.

The nurse took my blood pressure. It was 113 over 72. What could possibly scare me now? So, I met the doctor alone. This clean-cut, well-dressed man walked into the exam room with a big smile. "Hi! How are you today?"

"Great! How are you?"

"Good, thanks. So, why are you here today?" he asked. Was this guy kidding?

"I have cancer," I said, matter-of-factly, continuing the fake pleasantries.

"Oh, that's no big deal. We can take care of that. Let me look at your file," he said as he reviewed the pages and then got on his stool and wheeled over. He tells me to relax. Seriously? I'm spread like a frog pinned for dissection in biology class. If any woman is able to relax in this position, clearly they have bigger issues than cancer.

During the exam he said the cancer looked isolated. He said the tissue was soft and fleshy, which is always a good sign.

He pushed back his stool from the exam table. "This is no problem. I have patients that are complicated cases. I can fix this with a few snips. You're going to be just fine!"

He took a couple more samples for another biopsy and then scheduled me for an MRI. I like this guy. I like his disposition. Everything was going to be okay.

When my husband picked me up from the doctor's appointment I was excited. I told my husband how cool this guy was. I was not nervous, which scared my husband more than anything.

On the drive home my husband put his hand on my knee. "Are you okay?" he asked.

I laughed. "Yeah, I'm fine," I said as I smiled to myself.

"What's so funny?" he asked as I looked out the passenger side window.

"I'm going to write a book about this. I already have the title. It's funny. Do you want to hear it?" I asked.

"Sure."

I put my hands in the air as I told him the words. *"Thank God I Got Cancer, I'm Not a Hypochondriac Anymore!"* I said with a smile. I knew he would appreciate the genius that he married.

"That's not funny at all. Cancer isn't *funny*. How can you joke about that?" he asked with a scowl.

"Look, you know I've always been a hypochondriac. I have *literally* been training for this news my entire life. And now it's here. I have cancer. I feel like a superhero now. I'm invincible. My blood pressure was 113 over 72. I feel great. What could possible scare me now?"

He looked at me in disbelief.

"I'm going to put this in a book."

"Big surprise."

That was a big joke in my house and with extended family. When something funny or even something awful happens, everyone looks at me and says "put *that* in your next book." Writers do that as I'm sure you know. They write things about themselves. They are usually the protagonists in their books. But me, I'd never written a non-fiction book. This would be different.

That night I drove to Bonita Springs to see some friends of mine. One of them is hardcore into prayer. She shouted the cancer demon out of me as I watched with a raised eyebrow. Now, I do believe in miracles, but I have not been part of an actual exorcism before. It was a nice gesture and she was adamant about my cancer being cured…unless *I* did not believe it. Then it was my fault my cancer wasn't gone because I did not have enough faith. I exhaled and started wondering why I even bothered coming down here for this. I told her my doctor wanted to do surgery in two weeks. She kept saying, "Don't get the surgery. Wait for the healing."

Are you kidding me? Listen, God forbid you are diagnosed with cancer. No one should ever dictate to you what treatment options you should take. I'm certainly not a fan of "waiting for the healing." What if the healing God intends is by the hands of a surgeon? Then, I will have croaked, while "waiting for the healing."

My friend, Winnie, whose mother died of cancer, groaned when I told her about this. "Have the surgery!" she said. And she's churchy too. She didn't tell me to wait. She said it was ridiculous for anyone to say that if I'm not healed it's my fault because I don't believe. Now, I will say this: If I eat cheesecake every day and don't lose weight that *is* my fault. But, God allows us to go through things sometimes. I don't know why. Maybe "wait for the healing" knows. She seems to be an expert on all things God-related. What I do know is this, if your doctor says he or she can clean it up if they treat it now, I'd say to you, "*Don't* wait for the healing!"

My doctor asked me if I drank and I said no. He said that I should start drinking a glass of red wine every night. I told him that since I'd found out I had cancer it made me want to start drinking. Consult your doctor but this is something your oncologist will recommend. "Curing cancer one glass at a time" may not be good for everyone.

I cannot tell you how many people told me to send my thoughts about cancer and being healed "to the universe." What? I had never heard about this before.

Where I come from, we pray. The universe is lovely but I don't know what it has to do with my health. I did as they suggested and made my demand to the universe but I also prayed to God. Because, I know him...*personally.*

Your Doctor

If you or someone you know has cancer and they don't like their doctor, they need to get a new doctor right away. Every case may be different, but now because I had cancer, I have to go to the doctor every three months for the next five years. Your relationship with your cancer specialist will last longer than a Hollywood marriage. That's a lot of time to spend with someone that you don't like or trust. Consider this – you are literally putting your life in the hands of your doctor.

July 9

I'd never had an MRI before. I'd heard about them. I've known people that have had them. I had been able to evade them until now. The nurse put an IV in my arm.

Do you think I flinched? Not at all. I had cancer, baby. I wasn't about to let a little needle worry me! The MRI itself was fine. I just spent the forty-five minutes in prayer. Well, in prayer *and* at the beach. I found myself drifting to the beach in all my meditations of late. You'd be surprised how quiet it gets with a super loud machine when you're focused. I don't get focused very often. I was confident that I would be okay. The few people that did know were telling me to stay positive. This was an *actual* prayer I prayed:

"God, you know I'm not a positive or optimistic person. But I know I need to stay positive through this journey. So, please give me your peace and let me have hope beyond explanation…" and then I got worried. I was an award-winning comedy writer. Funny people are funny because they're *pessimists*! We would not have any material if we were positive. I knew I'd better put a caveat on that prayer… "But, not enough positive thoughts that it will hinder my ability to be funny or sarcastic. Amen."

I was doing so well in the MRI that the technician said over the microphone. "Are you okay in there?"

"Yeah, I'm great. Why? Am I moving too much?" I asked.

"No. You're perfect. You're not moving at all. I just wanted to make sure." Yup, suddenly, I'm a model patient. I pictured myself being at the beach. I was sitting in a chair with my toes in the sand and a drink in my hand. Yup, I wasn't in that machine at all. I was where waves were crashing and seagulls were squawking.

Just when I felt calm, the machine with all its beeps, chirps and whistles, this horrible tone came through that sounded like the words, "*DIE! DIE! DIE!*" in a deep and evil voice. Am I imagining that this machine sounds like it's telling me to DIE? General Electric built this machine. Aren't they still bringing things *to life*? I'd better start a dialogue in my head to change this now. There was a deep tone resonating over and over that sounded like Peter Frampton's talk box. If you don't know what I'm talking about, shame on you! If I'm going to be in this thing for another half hour I'd better get it in my head that it's saying, "LIVE! LIVE! LIVE!" in a sweet, high-pitched voice.

When it was over, the nurse took the IV out without me even squealing. My how I have grown. I drove myself home and started writing this book. I wanted to make sure I did it while it was fresh in my mind.

July 14

My husband and I waited for the doctor in his office. We looked around at all the awards this guy had. He had won 'Best Oncologist' so many times, I couldn't count all of the plaques by the time he came in. From a distance we heard someone singing "I'm Too Sexy." Of course, it was my doctor.

He gave us a big smile and shook our hands. "How are you guys doing?" he asked.

"Was that you singing 'I'm too sexy' in the hallway?" I asked.

He looked caught off-guard. "Maybe," he said hesitantly with a smile and one eyebrow raised. He pulled out the results of the biopsy and the MRI, along with a diagram of the female anatomy and explained what he wanted to do surgically. He said I also could do radiation but he talked me out of that pretty quickly when he described the side effects. My cancer was in stage 1 (b). The stages of cancer are determined by the size of the growth. I didn't know that until I had cancer and asked my oncologist. Thank God, it was caught early. And according to the MRI it looked isolated.

I looked at him thoughtfully and said, "I don't really want to have surgery, doc. Do I have another choice?"

He pretty much said I could have the surgery now…or eventually I'd *die*. I told him I was leaning towards the surgery. He said he thought I'd go that way.

Then my husband made the mistake of saying he saw Dr. Oz do a show about alternative medicine. Well, that sent my doctor off into a long dialogue about patients he's had that he could've saved but they'd opted for "alternative" treatments that not only proved ineffective but deadly. Especially when people purchased unapproved and untested medicine off the internet.

After he got that off his chest he showed me a diagram of what he was cutting out of me, which were parts I felt that I had really been using and gotten attached to over the years. I felt confident that this was the right guy for me. I asked the question I was sure others before me had asked, "Will I weigh less without that stuff?"

He just laughed.

When his staff tried to schedule the surgery the first available day was my birthday. I didn't think that was a good idea. So, I opted for the next available date, which was July 29. I was nervous that with the two-week recovery time I wouldn't be ready to pick up an award I'd won for my novel, "Mark Taylor's Checkered Past."

The awards ceremony was scheduled for August 8. I felt I would barely be making the three-hour drive from my house to Orlando. At least, I feared it wouldn't be a comfortable ride. I had to be there!

He assured me that I would be fine and I would be able to collect my award in person. After leaving the office with a stack of papers and a cancer magazine, I had to make a decision…and fast.

The next big decision I had to make was selecting who I was going to tell. Years ago when I stopped drinking I was surprised to learn that I did not have many friends left. This is a common occurrence with people who quit drinking. Because, whether you know it or not, you have a set of drinking friends and non-drinking friends. But you do not know who your real friends are until you stop drinking.

Guess what? The same thing happened when I told people I had cancer…and they're gone! Now some people got closer. They called and texted and asked what they could do. But many pulled away. And that's okay. I'm sure they don't know what to say unlike people who really care and say, "I'm sorry, I don't know what to say" and stick around anyway. Say goodbye to your fair-weather friends. That's not who you need when you have cancer anyway. Sometimes the things people say are more difficult to deal with than the cancer itself.

Warning: Stupid things you might hear from people:

- Can I have your jewelry? (I do have really good jewelry).
- I know someone who died from that. (Thanks, that's helpful).
- This is really inconvenient. (Oh, sorry. Cancer

wasn't taking appointments).

- At least you'll lose some weight! (Back at you, porky!)

- It's only Stage 1. (You will see later on how scary Stage 1 cancer can be!)

- OMG! Are you going to have that pelvic mesh put in that I keep seeing on those personal injury ads? (I really had someone ask me this. And my response was, "I'll have the life-saving surgery now and worry about the mesh afterwards!")

- You should go an alternative route! (Of course, these are people that have never had cancer and haven't been to med school. By all means, get another opinion but not a *stupid* one. I'm not saying you can't seek an alternative cure, but know that there are no guarantees. My oncologist told me he had patients that he could've cured that stopped treatment and wound up dying because they bought "alternative" medicine on the internet. There are scammers everywhere. Just do your due diligence. This is your *life* we're talking about.)

- You probably got cancer from your microwave!

Warning: Stupid things people may do:

- Cry
- High Drama (I actually had someone tell me that I was causing them stress by telling them I had cancer and they didn't need any more anxiety right now. I told her it was a good thing *she* wasn't the one who got cancer).
- Total Abandonment (not just friends, many relationships and marriages end during *and after* this crisis) You don't need people who aren't supportive. Now is the time to weed out the chaff.
- Gossip (this is really juicy and they thank God it's not *them*. But you will be a hot topic of discussion. I can almost hear the gasps right now).
- People will treat you like you're weak or

fragile. Don't take this crap from people! I didn't. I would even say, "Don't treat me like I'm sick just because I have cancer." Don't be afraid to speak up! Now don't confuse this point for "playing the cancer card." You are definitely going to want to do that. But, you should save that for when it will be most dramatic and impactful. It has more impact on someone when they don't know you have cancer. Enjoy it as their guilt sinks in. Really, you don't want to use it more than once. Make it count.

- Puppy dog eyes (do not allow people to pity you. In fact if they say, "Oh, I'm so sorry about your cancer," then you should find something physical on them and comment on it. For example, say, "And I'm sorry you wore those shoes with that shirt")

- There is a fringe element to many churches. Some people even made comments that I was living a sinful lifestyle that's why I got cancer. Don't listen to this crap. If everyone doing something sinful got cancer, everyone would have cancer. I wish that people who went to church would actually read their Bible. No one is fit to cast the first stone. That's too bad. There are a lot of people I'd like to throw rocks at.

You can get upset at the stupid things that people say and do. Or you can write them down and make money from it. I'd advise you to keep a journal. Other people's stupidity can equal comedy gold. Your own stupidity, however, should always be omitted from anything you write!

July 29

The day of the operation, I was feeling a lot of anxiety. I had a whole speech prepared for God. I was going to do what a lot of us do. I was going to bargain with Him. God, if you do this…then I'll do that. Ha ha ha! Why do any of us actually think we control anything? I had NO control over what was about to happen during surgery.

When I arrived there was a nice surgical nurse who checked me in. I had her laughing the whole time she was getting me prepped for surgery. She is what I call an "easy laugh." I love people like that because she laughed at everything I was saying. This is terrible encouragement for someone like me. By the time I was lying on the gurney and after I met the anesthesiologist another nurse said she was going to give me something to "relax" me. Oh good. I definitely need to relax!

My husband came in to see me off and as I was lying there, my heart monitor made a funny noise. Actually it was more like the sound of air raid drill. We looked at the monitor and it said "skipped a beat."

I tried to remain calm but I yelled, "Nurse! Nurse! Why did my heart skip a beat? That can't be good. I'm about to be put under."

She came over and laughed. "You're nervous. Sometimes our hearts skip a beat. You're going to be fine," she said as she reset the monitor.

"I thought that was just something writers say. Hearts actually skip a beat?" I asked.

"Yup, why don't I give you something else to make

you relax?" she said.

I didn't know it but I was only going to have a minute to tell my husband to remarry if anything should happen to me. He looked at me and sincerely said, "I wouldn't ever marry again. Just like I know you'd never marry again."

"Oh yes I would! And you should too. You're no good alone." I was not afraid. I mean, if something happened to me, I knew he'd never find anyone like me again. Ha! God broke the mold when he made me…very violently I'd imagine.

…And, goodnight nurse! I was out! The next thing I remember was my doctor waking me up and telling me everything went perfectly. They injected dye to make sure they got all the cancer out. Everything looked like it should. I was glad it did because I went night-night before I even got a chance to negotiate with God. Who was I kidding? Certainly, ahem, not God!

I had friends and family visit. I did not remember some of them even coming in. I was on some pretty strong stuff. I felt bad for Winnie. She told me this was the same oncology floor where her mom passed away.

Seeing me there brought back a lot of bad memories for her.

Things to take to the hospital:
- Cell phone (and charger)
- Slippers
- Bathrobe
- ID
- Insurance Card
- Music
- Snacks (if you're allowed)
- Books

DO NOT bring a mirror or make-up. You will look terrible so don't bother!

July 30

I was going home! Hard to believe, I had cancer one day, and then literally woke up and did not have it anymore. I was walking, able to keep food down and all my vitals were normal. The only thing was I could not drive for two weeks. Maybe some people would love that. But for me I was convinced it would be like imprisonment. My husband had to leave. Our Governor, Rick Scott, was coming down from Tallahassee to meet my husband and his partners on his job site. So, I did what any good wife did, I told him I'd call my mother and ask her to drive me home.

This upset him. He felt guilty – which is not usually an emotion that I let go of without milking a little bit – but I convinced him this may be a once-in-a-lifetime opportunity. He said, "But you had cancer!"

"Hopefully that too will be a once-in-a lifetime thing," I said. "Go… seriously," I prodded. As he walked out the door I stopped him. "Wait! Bring Governor Scott one of my books! He'll think it's funny since he's from Naples. Make sure you tell him I would have been there but I had cancer surgery." I know you probably think it's ridiculous that I would stoop so low. Oh well. Trust me, I didn't get where I'm at in life by not taking advantage of certain situations. Me an opportunist? Absolutely! It's not like it wasn't true!

I signed the book and he gave me a kiss and walked

out. I got the green light from the nursing staff and started getting dressed. I was going home. Yay! I was totally normal. Well, I had a catheter. That wasn't going to be pleasant but I was happy because I would be recovering at my home!

When the discharge nurse and my oncology nurse came in to check me out they went over the paperwork and aftercare instructions. And that's when I saw it...it was *terrifying*. It was the diagram of what the catheter's job was and how it was, uh, attached.

"Oh my God!" I squealed. "That's how that thing is staying up there?" to which they both laughed hysterically.

"How did you think it was staying up?" the discharge nurse asked.

"I don't know. NASA technology? I thought it was orbiting me or something. That's *disgusting!* And now that diagram is burned into my brain!" I closed my eyes and opened them. *"No! I can still see it,"* I said, to which they again laughed.

We were almost done with the paperwork when the nurse wanted to make sure I knew not to have sex. I just looked at her with a long pause.

"Seriously? That's deeply disturbing to me that you have to drive that home. I'm at 'no vacancy' status right now. People are freaks!"

"Yes. Yes, they are."

God knows, I'm no prude. But seriously, people, that's nasty!

My mom came to get me and as I was wheeled away, I told the hospital staff I hoped I would never see them again! But I knew I had to write the hospital a letter commending them on their outstanding staff. From the girl who brought me my meals with a smile and small talk to the nursing staff and doctors doing their rounds – this hospital was outstanding.

They transformed a potentially terrifying experience into a good one. I was confident that this journey could not be kept to myself. I did not want someone else to go through this without knowing what to expect.

My husband said the Governor was very nice and noticed the dedication to my book was to the staff at Hazelden in Naples. And like any good politician, he promised that he would read it. He remarked that he was a big reader and liked humor. You never know. I can tell when someone thinks I'm funny in person…they laugh. But, like email or texting, you don't know how someone is interpreting your written words. And I know not everyone has my sense of humor. Too bad. The world would be a better place! Humor has always been a great coping mechanism in my family but that is irrelevant. My husband didn't get much time to talk with the Governor anyway, just enough to give him my book. And really, I'm just trying to get the word out about my books.

I had so many people coming in and out of my house that I contemplated tying a big bow on the tube of my catheter. It was just…there. The hospital staff didn't want me continually getting up and down so they gave me a huge, conspicuous bag to collect pee until I could get up and use the "to-go" version. I know this is going to anger some people but for me the catheter was worse than the whole cancer process. I mean, all I did was show up. The doctors and nurses did all the work. That's so typical of me. I have a problem and other people clean it up. Thanks, everyone!

Wi-Fi was laying down with me on the sofa. She only

left my side to go to the bathroom and eat. She had never done that before. She was also playing with my catheter every time I got up to go to the bathroom or eat. I don't know why she found it fun to chase my tubing. She has a sick sense of humor!

My friends Winnie and Joy came over with dinner for a few nights. I was so glad. All my husband can make is eggs and chili and obviously that would get old very fast. The good news was I didn't have to cook. People had offered to bring us meals for the next two weeks. The bad news was I have a huge ego and think I'm a great cook. Yet, everyone else's food tasted so much better than mine. Oh well, maybe they'll hold a cooking class for me when I'm well!

For those who couldn't visit, the flowers, plants and get-well cards started coming in. It was nice to feel loved. Not by everyone though. There were certainly key family members and "friends" who knew about my situation and:

a) didn't care or…

b) were too distraught to reach out (and yet I'm the one who was diagnosed with cancer)

Some people do not know what to say. All they have to do is stick a card in the mail or tell you that they're thinking about you. If you have any suspicion that someone does not care about you it will be confirmed when you have cancer. It's okay. It makes it easier to revise your will! You will be surprised by who flees and who stays and rallies around you in this time of need. It happens to all cancer patients. And if so-and-so wasn't nice to you before you got cancer, don't think they're going to be nice after.

July 31

It was a slow day. I am taking pain meds, but they're not helping.

August 1
8:00 a.m.

According to the hospital's discharge papers I'm supposed to poop today. If I don't, I'll have to start taking constipation medicine. I started to think about all the food in my body that I haven't pooped out yet. I'm starting to feel gross and bloated but it's probably psychological. At least I'm not in any pain. I stopped taking my pain meds because I don't need them. It hurts to laugh, cough and sneeze.

10:00 p.m.

There's blood in my catheter. That can't be good. I called my doctor's office. The doctor on call was so nice and he called back me in four minutes. He said my surgical site was irritated and that a few little flakes with blood are normal and nothing to be concerned about.

August 2

I have a lot of gas today. I reflect to my last meal before the surgery (which was my birthday dinner). I wonder about my poor colon and the birthday steak I ate. I curse you, red meat! I curse you and…I love you! My stomach feels so heavy. I wonder how much food your body can store before it kills you. I'm not a bear!

August 3

I drank cherry magnesium citrate to get this party started. I thought the catheter was the worst part of this experience. It's not. Lots of gurgling. No pooping.

August 4
8:00 a.m.

Called my doctor's office. They said take a pain pill and a laxative. They advised me to relax and let it fall out naturally. God help me if poop ever falls out of me *unnaturally*.

1:00 p.m.

Laying on the sofa, staring at the ceiling, watching the fan spin. Got on Facebook. Fantasized about posting status update of "I pooped!" Of course I never would really post that. I didn't tell many people about the cancer – never mind not pooping! But I was alarmed that the ones that did know kept texting, asking if I pooped with the little turd emoticon. I actually had someone ask if I'd had a good bowel movement lately. Honestly, that might've been funny if they weren't serious. Classy! Call me old-fashioned but I've never asked anyone about their bowels.

August 5

My, my, how my prayers have changed in a week. I went from saying, "God, don't let me die on the operating table" to "God, if you really liked me you'd let me poop!"

August 6

Finally on day seven, I pooped. And it was a massive amount. I actually worried that I put a burden on the septic tank. The other good news, I must weigh at least ten pounds less now.

August 7

My follow-up appointment with my oncologist's office was today. I look at the appointment card. I don't want to be late! Wait a minute. The card says "catheter check" not removal. They said it would only have to be in for seven days. It must be an oversight. Surely, they're removing this today. I hate it. When it's empty it follows me around the house like a bad dog. I haven't even left the house in a week! I don't want to go out with this thing. There are straps that wrap around my thigh with a bag. It's not cool. It's not like I have a thigh holster and I'm packing, just waiting to blow a bad guy away. What I have is a urine grenade. How would I intimidate anyone with that? This sucks! And, to make matters worse, I'm driving to Orlando tomorrow to pick up my award for my book. I can't have a catheter. Please, God. No!

So, I go to the doctor's office positive that this thing was coming out. They shoot liquid in my bladder to test my reaction. I should have to pee – instantly. And then I'm commanded to do something else that repulses me, sit on a toilet. Ew. A public toilet? Without a bleach bomb? Ugh. So, I sit there and sit there, and sit there. The nurse calls to me, "How are you doing in there?" she asks.

"I can't pee!" I shout out in a sorrowful voice. I'm in agony. I'm not peeing and I'm not peeing on a public toilet that I didn't get to wipe first. Ugh. I sat there thinking about me waddling across the stage with my catheter and bag o'urine. I sit with my left hand under my chin and my right hand filled with a wad of toilet paper, anticipating even a trickle.

I hear this voice in my head, "You're lucky, some people have to wear these every day of their lives." Oh, shut up, I say to myself.

The nurse walks in, which is new to me. I don't even allow my husband see me on the toilet at home. Some things are just better left behind closed doors. "How's it going?" she asks.

"Not good. Is my bladder broken? I have somewhere really important to go tomorrow. I can't have this thing in!"

The nurse looked at me and I don't know if she was trying to make me feel better or worse when she said, "You know, I had a woman a lot younger than you that had to keep it in for six weeks." Six weeks? Ugh. I'm screwed.

So, there I was, a few minutes later, getting another catheter put in. And, it hurt. The first time, I was unconscious and if you have a choice, knocked out is the way to go!

I walked out of there with a funny little walk. This catheter tube was hard and not flexible. It hurt. Not to mention, my stomach was starting to get bloated again. I wondered how bad I'd look at the awards banquet.

We packed the bags and left the house for Orlando. Without using my brain, I told my husband we should take my vehicle. Why is that a big deal? I drive a manual transmission. He does not. I *like* driving a manual transmission. He does not. Coincidently, I do not like *him* driving a manual transmission, especially with me in my condition. What a hurky, jerky, terrible ride. Mental note to myself: I am never buying him a vintage sports car.

August 8

I look awful! The gown I bought doesn't fit. I am so bloated, I look pregnant. I should've shopped in the maternity section to begin with. So there I was in Marshalls, two hours before the awards banquet, trying to find anything that would fit over my post-cancer speed bump. It was a speed bump. It was definitely slowing me down. The only dress I could find was just okay looking. It was blue, green and white. It was almost a convincing knock-off of a Tommy Hilfiger design. It had weird little shapes that resembled fish scales and it was fitted. It did fit over the speed bump so I was buying it.

At the banquet I texted one of my friends and warned her to look for the pregnant mermaid. Oh well, I'd just blame cancer. I knew some of the other writers there. Not everyone knew my condition. I certainly wasn't my energetic, bubbly self and I did wind up revealing what was going on. There were a lot of people asking me what was happening because some of them heard I wasn't in good health. Aside from my appearance I was actually feeling okay. I was just really puffy.

I kept having to go to the bathroom and empty my pee bag, which wasn't a huge deal, except for these things:

a) I had to stand *facing the toilet* and lift my dress to

empty my bag.

b) Anyone looking under the stalls can see this and hear someone *"peeing."*

c) This is not how a *woman* typically empties her bladder.

d) I may not look like a woman right now because I have my grandfather's eyebrows and my grandmother's mustache. Yup, I've officially let myself go. Stupid cancer.

e) I wonder if any of this is even relevant anymore because of all the controversy over unisex bathrooms. I guess in the long run, I still "identified" with being a woman. Maybe a Neanderthal, but at least a female one.

At the end of the night, I collected my medal and went back to the resort where we were staying. Tomorrow, we would make arduous journey back to Fort Myers…in a *five-speed*.

August 9

We had breakfast at a famous buffet restaurant chain. Like I didn't feel like a fat enough pig. The good news for me was even with my huge, swollen speed bump I was still way smaller than their average customer. I got depressed watching the large customers with their large plates filled with simple carbs. I wondered why *I* got cancer when I had eaten reasonably healthy for my adult years. I wanted to shout it from the sneeze guards, "Low carb, high protein, people!" But I think it would have fallen on deaf ears.

August 10

I find out another person I know just got diagnosed with cancer. I offer what advice I can but their prognosis is not optimistic as mine was. They have a more complicated and advanced cancer.

August 13

"Wait for the healing" rears her head. She texted me and I knew the courteous thing was to call her and tell her how I was doing. When she expressed her disappointment in me having surgery over "waiting for the healing" I told her that I know for a fact that it's not God's plan to heal everyone.

"How do you know?" she asked.

"Because there are a lot of *dead* people!" I said.

I'm not an evil person. But, I did think about her appendix. Now, I didn't want her to *die*. I just wanted her doctor to tell her that they needed to remove her appendix immediately because her life depended on it. That way, when she was being wheeled away on the gurney I could shout, "Wait for the healing." I know that's immature. At this point of the book, are you really surprised?

August 14

I went back to my doctor for another "catheter check." I had a different nurse this time. This lady was funny and she meant business. She said she was going to keep shooting saline in my bladder until I peed. I expressed concern that I just didn't feel like I had to pee. She explained that my bladder is in a different position now because of the surgery. I didn't know that. Before the surgery, I felt like my bladder was in a really good place. She suggested I rock back and forth gently. She told me I would have to learn how to pee again. She convinced me I did have to pee even if it didn't feel like it. I had déjà vu when I said, "God, if you really liked me you'd let me *pee*!" I kept thinking about Niagara Falls and within five minutes I peed. Thank God! I could wear short skirts again. Who knew I'd be grateful for something simple, like sitting down to pee! But, I still did not *feel* like I had to pee even though I did.

August 15

I researched this thing called a "Squatty Potty." I bought one from Bed, Bath & Beyond. They help people with bladder (and other) bathroom issues. I highly recommend one after surgery.

August 23

I contacted my editor and told him I was sending my manuscript over. After my dramatic bout with cancer my book was done! That night, I told my husband to pray for two other people we knew that were about to start chemo. *Those poor suckers.* I'm so lucky I didn't have to get chemo.

This is where my book originally ended, with me being cancer-free. Yay! I even called my editor and said my manuscript was on the way. It would be a cute little booklet on cancer. I should say it *was* a little booklet.

August 25

I went back to my oncologist for my first post-op visit. I was confident that everything would be fine. Until, he gave me an awkward smile said, "Let's go talk in the conference room," as he walked with a manila file folder. It's been my experience in life that whenever a man says he wants "to talk," it doesn't ever end well. He opened up the file and my husband came in and sat down. "So, the operation went perfectly. And, the preliminary pathology report looked clear. Except..."

This is the point where I wanted to stick my fingers in my ears and say repeatedly, "I'm not listening to you," while I rocked back and forth. But I didn't. I adjusted positions in my chair and braced myself for more bad news.

"I removed seventeen of your lymph nodes during the surgery, but the pathology report came back showing the cancer had spread to two of them. There are still cancer cells on the lymph trail. Three years ago, we didn't even have this technology. By the time we would've found out it was spreading to the other lymph nodes you would've been in real trouble. We are going to get you started with chemo and radiation to kill the cells now."

I asked, "Are you sure I'm not getting enough radiation from my iPhone? Because, I'm on that *a lot*." And that's when my doctor gave me "the look."

"You're going to have to see another doctor in our practice. He's a radiation expert. He'll evaluate your case and come up with the proper course of treatment," he added.

"Okay," I said, very calmly. I looked at my husband. He was not handling it as well as I was. I know God is the ultimate comedian because the nurse told me I will have to get lab work done every week during chemo. He's so funny. More needles.

I told my doctor that this sucked because I had already turned my manuscript in to my editor. He said he had another patient writing a book as well. He thought John Goodman would be a good actor to play him, which I thought was strange since my doctor is a handsome man who's in good shape.

On the ride home my husband said, "I don't know why he wouldn't want Bradley Cooper to play him."

I said, "I'll tell you what, as a patient, I would *not* want to look down and see Bradley Cooper there."

"I just meant in the *movie* version," he said.

So much for people telling me to, "Send it to the universe." I sent my wishes for healing to the universe. This is what I learned...*the universe is a dog and I am its fire hydrant.*

Unfortunately, this was right after Jimmy Carter had made an announcement that he had terminal cancer. I texted my mom that my cancer had spread and I would need chemo and radiation. I told her my prognosis was good. Hours went by and she didn't text me back. However, she dropped by unannounced and when I opened the door, I asked her if she read the text.

"Yeah, your cancer spread...*like Jimmy Carter*!" she wailed as she came into my house.

"Mom, he's terminal. I'm going to be fine," I said. Geez. And everyone thinks *I'm* dramatic. So after we talked for a little while, I tried to convince her that this was really a way better story for the book anyway. She didn't appreciate that. No one wants to read about a quick little surgery to clean up cancer. Now the book would have some real meat. She just folded her arms and gave me "the look." Of course we find out later on, by some miracle, he's cancer-free.

I have to say it again with a small change. When it comes to being healed, sometimes God uses radiation technicians and chemo nurses to save your life.

August 26

I cried at a Kleenex commercial and I didn't even have a tissue. How ironic. Cancer has made me so soft. It's really pathetic. No one can know I have functioning tear ducts.

My friend asked me if my doctor was going to run a CT scan. I didn't know. I asked her why. She told me her mom had abdominal pains for years and no one could figure out why. They gave her a CT scan and it came back clear. When they did exploratory surgery, they found stage IV cancer. She died two weeks later. It made me think that catching cancer early enough to treat it may just be dumb luck.

August 27

Someone who knew me stopped me when they saw me out and asked me about my condition. I was wearing sunglasses indoors and didn't take them off because I was a wreck. I told her it had spread even though my prognosis was still good, then I looked at my watch and said, "Now, if you'll excuse me, I am doing charity work this morning. I have to go help the *less fortunate*," I added before cackling out loud. Now, I just want to make clear that I don't do a lot of charity work. I'm not bragging about doing a lot. I guess I just bragged about *not* doing a lot. I help others when I have writer's block. I guess I'm selfish in my charity work then. Whenever people see me doing charity work they ask how many community service hours until I meet my requirement. Apparently, many people my age don't do charity work voluntarily.

August 30

It has become painfully obvious that some people are real idiots and don't actually think before they speak. Also, everything is magnified at this point. I marvel at my powers of observation. I notice what a wuss everyone else is. With every burn from toast or static shock resulting from doing laundry, every little squeal of pain from people around you is annoying. You wonder if you're the strongest person on earth. You certainly note that you are the least whiney.

The Next Round of "Stupid Things People Say."

- Someone found out I was having chemo said, "Oh no, are you going to lose your hair?" I wonder with cancer looming over me why someone would think I give a rat's butt about being bald? I'm trying to outrun the Grim Reaper here. Please people, use some common sense.

- Radiation is going to give you cancer. Hello? I already *have* cancer. Duh. Let's fight fire with fire then.

- Big Pharma is trying to poison you with chemo. What? They're trying to prolong my life. So, think what you want but don't tell every stupid opinion you have to the cancer patient. Especially, when YOU have not been through cancer treatment.

My sister (who thinks she is psychic) flies down from Massachusetts for moral support. Mine or hers, I don't fully know. I secretly wonder why her crystal ball did not tell her that I still had cancer. For that matter, it didn't tell her I had it either. Maybe it's broken.

August 31

My sister asks me to go to a crystal bowl healing with her. I own several pieces of Waterford and they have not healed me yet. If there was one company I would think could cure me – it would be them. I do not know what this "bowl healing" nonsense is but I warned her that it was just going to wind up in my book.

September 1

I met my radiation team. Lucky for me, they're amusing too. My husband asked how the cancer spread into the lymph nodes when it was only in stage 1. We then learned it was more advanced than they thought and what was revealed in the MRI. The doctor commented that they never know what they'll find until they "look under the hood."

The CT scan

This was nothing! It's hardly even worth mentioning, the

tech has you lie down, they run the scan and you're done. Five minutes, tops! I start thinking it's funny when I hear people mention that I'm "battling" cancer. *I'm just sitting there!* It's not my battle. It's up to people working in radiation and chemo now.

A Permanent Reminder of Cancer

I made my mom a lot of promises when I was a young woman. I actually kept one of them. I never got a tattoo…until now. Today, I got three. The same person who ran the CT gave them to me. It wasn't my choice. You have to get them when you have radiation. It's so the technician can line up the laser beams at the same spots every time.

I remember that The Fantastic Four got their super powers because they were exposed to radiation. I was excited. If there was a time in my life I thought I'd have a shot at getting my super powers, it was now!

7:00 p.m.

Remember how I agreed to go with my sister to her crystal bowl healing? Tonight was the night. As we drove, I reiterated how I didn't like psychics and thought they were frauds, which upset my sister, because remember, she thinks she *is* one. When we get to the shop I'll call "Unicorn Headquarters," (because I don't want to encourage anyone to go to the real place) my sister tells the head priestess that we are siblings and this makes the Elvira-wannabe ecstatic. Now she "knows" something about us that will help her cold read later.

She tells us to take a spot on the floor – like animals! We find two spots next to each other. I can't help but chuckle out loud when I look at the sea of tie-dye, gypsy-skirted believers. I'm dressed like I'm in town for a Republican convention. I lay down and someone passes me a lucky stone to hold onto while I'm meditating. I laugh again and say thanks as I pass the bowl to some other sucker. My sister reminds me to be "open to the spirit guides." I just look at her. I look around the room and think what a racket this is. Then the Princess of Darkness comes to the room and says she's going to start the healing process.

I'm so excited. I can't wait to tell my doctor that I'm cured! I'll have to buy him a black robe and some sage. Too bad he wasted all those years in med school.

She begins by lighting several candles and then starts chanting. I try and close my eyes, but I get distracted by what looks like the Grim Reaper holding his scythe. Argh! Scary! Never mind. That was just the lady stirring her bowls. Hey, it was dark in there. After I hear all the same sounds as were in my MRI, the session is over. She thanks the crowd and just as I was getting up and shaking the fairy dust off my clothes, the Princess of Darkness points to me and says, "Wait…you!"

Oh crap, she's looking at me. I point to myself and say, "Me?" And she shook her head in slow-motion.

"I have a message for you," she says and I hear a collective "oooh" from the believers who are now all staring at me.

I hope it's a just phone message from my husband.

"What?" I ask with a snarl of skepticism so she knows I'm not "open" to hearing it.

"I have a message from your father from the other side," she says with a slick smile.

"The other side of…*town*?" I ask with a smirk.

She panics, "Oh, your father hasn't crossed over?"

I look at my watch, "He may be crossing over the Caloosahatchee Bridge right now," I say with a smirk. "He's on his way home from work."

She's clearly startled. "Uh, oh, well, he wanted me to tell you he's proud of you," she said quickly.

"*Okay*," I say with a chuckle to her as I asked my sister, "You ready now?"

When we get out to the car, I prod my sister. "Surely you can't believe in this crap after that?"

"Obviously she wasn't a *real* psychic," she says.

I exhale, "Obviously," I say as I roll my eyes. I told my sister we should call my dad on the way home just to make sure the "spirit guides" knew something we didn't. He laughed at the whole thing and said he couldn't wait to read about it in my book.

September 10
3:30 p.m.

My first radiation treatment went something like this: I

signed in and was told to use the "Employees Only" door and then go to another waiting room. There, I was to put on an ugly pink gown and strip down to my underwear. Then, I wait for the radiation technicians to call me back. When I got back there, I told them my name and birthdate. I was then ushered into a room where the cradle that was made for me at my CT scan was pulled out and placed on the bed of the radiation machine. I was then told to lie down and they would position me as to line up the laser beams with my tattoos.

As I lie there wondering when my panic attack would happen (it didn't though because I was too busy thinking about what I was going to write about here for you) the techs roll down my panties and I make the mistake of looking to the right at the 35" monitor hanging from the ceiling. Hello, kitty! Apparently, they have a camera right on my exposed crotch to make sure the alignment is correct. The camera is used later on to make sure no one is actually having a panic attack because you're in the air about five feet off the ground.

Yup, I'm glad I didn't become an actress. I didn't appreciate looking bigger on camera. It was like a bad fifties sci-fi movie where the audience can't really decipher what kind of monster is on the screen. I could picture movie-goers with their popcorn, saying to each other, "What *is* that?" The techs then gave me a little pat on my arm and told me they'd be back in ten minutes after the program had run.

I have some advice for radiation patients. Netflix has "2001: A Space Odyssey." You need to watch it. Surprisingly, if you put yourself in the main character's place you will have many of the same emotions in radiation as you have watching this flick, such as:

- Is my breathing really this loud?
- I wish I didn't feel so isolated.
- Why is everything white in here?
- I don't understand what's happening.
- Why are there so many annoying beeps and chirps?
- God help me. When is this going to end?
- Is my heart rate faster than normal? It feels faster.
- Why is that red light on the wall staring at me? Is it really controlling everything?
- Why is there a baby floating around here? Just

kidding. That definitely shouldn't happen in radiation!

I love science fiction. If you don't like it, you will have a problem with radiation. I seriously encourage you to check this movie out. If you can make it through the movie, you'll be fine during radiation!

The fact that you will have radiation everyday will not make it easier because you get used to it. Some days, I pretended that it was me and not Luke Skywalker delivering the final strike to the Death Star. That machine just keeps rotating and I deal with things by letting my mind go somewhere else. I did ask if I could bring music. I strongly recommend doing that. Now, be reasonable. Don't listen to hard rock. You should listen to something calming. Download a few Dave Koz songs. Everyone should have sax in radiation. I also listened to what I call my sister's "hippie chimes." They are calming for most people. Don't listen to anything that's going to raise your heart rate because trust me, you'll hear and feel your heart beat no matter how loud your headphones are!

There is one thing I want to make you aware of.

Depending on who is running the machine that day, you will have the same treatment but it may be in a different order. After having treatments the same time every day you get to know the way the machine rotates. One day you may notice that the machine is rotating in the opposite direction. You are still getting the same dose. If you are concerned with a change in your routine, stay on the table! You are not at ground level while under treatment. When the treatment is over you can then ask your technician.

September 11

I pull into the cancer center's parking lot and notice a city tourist bus and laugh. I walk up to the receptionist and say, "There's a huge city tourist bus in the parking lot."

She seems surprised. "There is?"

"Yeah, I hope the driver has cancer or that's the worst tour ever!" We both laugh.

On my way up to her desk I passed a guy who was around my age. He was smoking a cigarette in front of the "No Smoking" sign. And, he was hacking. I thought to myself, I hope he's not here for lung cancer.

Before radiation I have to get blood work for chemo. This is going to happen every Friday since I have chemo on Mondays. They are checking white blood cell count, red blood cell count and kidney function. I watch the nurse stick me and draw my blood. I confess that I used to pass out but I'm cured of that stupid fear now.

As the treatments progress, if your numbers go down you may have to skip a treatment.

The whole thing becomes overwhelming to me. I am the type of person who does not even take acetaminophen when I have a headache. I hate medicine. I have to be really sick to use it. This though, this is a lot for me to take.

September 14

You should always take time to read the posters in the elevator. Some are very informational. Some are just laughable. Like this one, "Have you experienced anxiety as a result of your cancer spreading? If so, there's a research study for patients who are experiencing anxiety due to their cancer spreading." Really? Show me a patient who doesn't have anxiety from that!

I go to the chemo floor and check in. They take me back, I get weighed and then they walk me to a recliner. I sit down and a nursing assistant comes over and asks with a smile if I'd like a warm blanket. Another nurse greets me and takes my blood pressure and temperature. They ask my name and birthdate. The nurse then explains what is going to happen.

She is going to give me a two-hour drip of saline. I will have to pee 200 ML out or they can't give you chemo because it's so toxic, you have to prove you can pee it out before they even put it in your drip. They can't use your elbow or wrist veins because chemo will do permanent joint damage if it leaks. So, they have to find a vein on the inside or outside of your forearm. She asks if I want a certain drug. I told her I didn't know what that was. She said it will give me a feeling of euphoria. I said, "Sure, I'll order the full party package." She snickered. Then comes the sedative, anti-nausea medicine and magnesium. Next is chemo. After you pee, you have to flush twice, again, because of the medicine's toxicity.

After chemo, you get more saline to help you flush it through your system. Keep in mind, I still have no feeling when I have to pee anymore. So all of my bathroom trips are pre-emptive. Picture this with me attached to the IV and having to wheel it to the bathroom. Oh, and the best part? Guess who I get seated next to? Remember the smoker from last week? Yeah, he's there. After we chat, he confesses that he's there for lung cancer. It's so hard not be judgmental especially since I see people missing appointments because their insurance company denied their claims. It makes me sick.

On that note, I'd like to just say that we have Blue Cross and Blue Shield and they paid everything without a fight. We've had other insurance companies who argued over paying for annual health exams. People have enough to worry about when getting cancer treatments. No one should ever be denied treatment, especially if a chain smoker can get it.

The dietician came over and reviewed my diet plan. Because chemo makes you constipated and radiation makes you have diarrhea, she thinks I may be okay because the side effects will cancel each other. She found me a week after my first treatment and gave me some recipes and diet tips. She tells me that they do not want me to lose weight until the treatment is over in six weeks. When you're going through something terrible like this, it makes a world of difference when people act like they care. Everyone at this place goes above and beyond.

Some things to note during chemo treatment:

- You will need to use baby shampoo.
- You may not be able to dye your hair.
- You may not be able to style your hair with hot irons.
- If you lose your hair, it will probably grow back differently. If it was straight, it may be curly and vice versa. Someone told me their hair grew back an entirely different color! I've always had curly hair. After having chemo, it's now straight. Also, my hair grew back a different color – gray. I'm sure it's age-related but I blame cancer anyway!
- You will need to use a soft toothbrush and brush every day and night.

- You may get mouth sores. You should gargle with warm salt water a few times a day.

- You will get cold in the chemo room. They are putting cool liquids in your blood.

- You will have to flush your toilet twice every time you use the bathroom. Make sure you keep your toilet seat closed as to not poison your pets, if they drink out of the bowl.

- You may experience memory problems. It's called, "chemo brain." If you're absent-minded and have a short attention span like me maybe no one will notice! This problem with memory recall may last beyond your treatments.

- No more deep tissue massages. Sorry! That is not really a problem for me because I do not like strangers touching me. However, for those of you who *do* like strangers touching you, you will have to go to a massage therapist who specializes in oncology massage. Because of chemo (this also applies to radiation patients) you're more likely to develop (DVT) Deep Vein Thrombosis. Cancer changes *everything*.

- If you have a maid, they will have to use your broom, vacuum and mop. You can't take a chance of bringing someone else's germs into your home. It may be a good time to impose a no-shoe policy too, for your guests. I didn't want to say anything but your guest are dirty!

My chemo nurse sat down and talked about the possible side effects I could experience. She asked me if the radiation department informed me that my skin may get darker. And she said I will probably lose weight. I perked up. "Wait a minute. I'm going to be thinner and tan? I'm gonna be gorgeous when I get out of here!"

She laughed and said probably not.

The thing that was so surprising to me about chemo was that everyone looked like me in radiation. Not in chemo. Even the black folks looked white.

The deli downstairs made lunch for all the patients and put them in a cute little box that looked like a basket. After lunch I took a nice relaxed nap. I was as peaceful as Sleeping Beauty. She was a drooler too. A lot of people don't know that because it was omitted from the original story.

I was peaceful. That is, until I woke up to a panicked nurse who didn't know why my blood pressure was only 95 over 54. My nurse had gone to lunch and there was another nurse taking my blood pressure. So she called another nurse over and I leaned over to my husband and said, "See, I have super-low blood pressure and I don't even care. This stuff is awesome!" Turns out, the sedative they gave me was not only fun but also dropping my blood pressure, which is normal. However, this nurse didn't know that and was startled by it.

September 15

The radiation technicians asked me how I felt after my first chemo treatment. I was fine. They informed me that sometimes it takes a couple of days before I feel it.

September 16

They were right. This morning I woke up and my legs were red and hot. I felt nauseous but not that bad. I did not want to take the medicine they prescribed me for nausea because I was up late last night watching TV and there was an ad from a personal injury attorney. It said, "Did you or someone you love take blah, blah, blah while pregnant and have a two-headed baby?" Okay, I don't have a uterus anymore but I have to wonder, if it's producing two-headed babies then what will it do to me? I just decided I would eat every time I felt that way. That sounds like a good plan, right? Yup. I can't see how that would end badly.

Today is the first day I begin my weekly visit to the doctor's office after radiation. I meet with my physician's assistant. He asks how I am feeling and if I am having any side effects of the radiation or chemo. I tell him I am having minor nausea, but it's nothing I can't handle. He mentions I may notice my skin getting a little darker in the area being radiated and my hair will fall out. He wanted to make sure I wasn't experiencing any burning or dry skin in the radiated areas. I wasn't. He said unless I had any questions I was free to go. I told him that this was a boring visit and that I got all nervous for nothing. He smiled and said if I had any questions, I didn't need to wait until my next appointment. He gave me his business card and told me I could call him anytime, even weekends.

My Diet

For radiation they recommended restricting red meat. They said legumes were the perfect food. They said I had to be careful with fruits and veggies aggravating my stomach, which will be sensitive due to the area that was being radiated. Green, leafy vegetables are a must. They also recommend pudding, popsicles and broths.

On the other hand, for chemo they recommended 3-4 servings of red meat a week to keep my red blood cell count up. I had to restrict highly fibrous foods to avoid stomach agitation. Crackers and toast just became my new best friends.

This diet was no problem for me. I love red meat. I dated a vegetarian once. *Once.* When my husband is feeling amorous, he doesn't waste money on flowers, he makes beef brisket.

A word to vegetarians:

1. I'm sorry you have cancer.
2. I'm sorry you're a vegetarian.

You will have to discuss healthy diet options during your treatment. You have to keep your protein levels high!

Diabetics will also have to consult a dietician for healthy food choices during treatment.

As far as eating healthy, you should mix turmeric, garlic salt and black pepper. For some reason, when these three are combined they are like a super herb. Be warned, if you cook with them, your food will produce a fluorescent yellow liquid! But, I eat this blend at least once a day. If you cook/bake with it and put an Herbes de Provence blend (savory, thyme, basil, rosemary, fennel and lavender) with it, it will hide the strong turmeric taste.

Curry is another great spice to diminish the turmeric. Greens are an absolute must every day. I would also recommend switching to a low-carb, high protein diet. I always try and eat non-genetically modified foods, paired with a gluten-free diet. Please consult your doctor and be open to modifying your diet. Eat to live! But by all means, eat chocolate! It's good for you anyway!

September 18

I didn't listen to music today. That was a mistake because my mind really goes to strange places. I wondered what would happen if I put some popcorn kernels in my underwear? Then I started laughing. What if they actually popped? I bet that would look a little strange to the radiation technicians. It's not every day someone gets a popcorn erection. Well, at least I hope it's not. Then I watched the machines arms rotate and started thinking this must be what a rotisserie chicken feels like.

September 21

My second round of chemo. It was pretty uneventful. The nurse took my final blood pressure reading for the day and my husband asked her if she'd take his. She did. It was 151 over 96. I asked him if he had to pee. He just gave me "the look."

September 23

If you can walk or do light exercise, I recommend it. There are studies about cancer patients reducing their side effects by doing yoga. To be honest, I prefer "being one" with someone else. And I love pretzels but I don't like becoming one. To make it more annoying, I can't stand the chanting crap. You'll just have to find a yoga place you like. I prefer walking but that's me. I did check out a couple of yoga DVDs from the library but I turned the volume down.

You don't even look sick

I'm so sick of people telling me "You look so healthy." They seem disappointed. I want to ask them if they'd feel better if I looked like an extra from "The Walking Dead." If you have to work outside your home, I feel really bad for you. You are going to be exhausted. Cancer is not just a physical battle. You will have days that are very emotional. I still get choked up talking about it. I probably will never get over the emotions from my cancer experience. But know that you are in this for a reason. I believe it's to help other people.

I made friends at radiation. That happens easily because the appointments are the same time every day. While you're waiting for treatment, you wind up hearing and sharing very similar stories with the other patients. You find yourself talking and laughing with people who can identify with what you're going through. One friend said when she was done with her treatments, she wasn't going to tell other people she had cancer. I told her that it's her story but there may be a time she needs to share it to help someone else. I never got angry at God as some people do. I knew right away when I got cancer that it was so I could write a book about it.

People are going to want to help. I know you're tough and you feel like there's nothing anyone can do. You should tell people that if they could make you dinner one night that it would be really helpful. I had so many people bring me meals and I am very grateful that they did. You are going to underestimate how taxing the treatments are on you. Ask for help! If you need something from the store, ask someone to get it. Listen, people can't do much. Maybe have a close friend take you to treatment. Some of them are curious. I was never close to anyone who had cancer. I had no idea what happened in treatment. People will genuinely want to help you. Cancer is no time for pride!

I received many cards from friends and family. People were telling me that they were putting my name on prayer lists at their churches. I even had people who didn't go to church praying for me. I can't tell you how good it felt to have a thousand people praying for me. The good news was most of them were praying *I'd live*.

I really recommend wearing make-up and doing your hair (consult your doctor first!) For the last five years, I have used Origins make-up. I strongly recommend it. You don't need to be adding extra toxicity to your body with other brands of make-up. I wanted to look normal. You don't want to look sick. God forbid! People are so obnoxious. You know how when you're sick you get pale? I'm so pale already I was worried I'd be invisible.

Oh, maybe *that* was my super power!

September 28

My chemo nurse asked if I was having side-effects. I told her that I had a little nausea but it was nothing I couldn't handle. She asked me if I was taking the medicine they prescribed. I told her that I wasn't. Then I told her about the ad I saw. She looked at me and started laughing. "We've been putting that in your chemo drip every week. Don't be a hero. Just take your medicine!"

She did recommend that I get my hair cut. The extra weight of my long hair was putting stress on my roots. She recommended that I get it cut before it falls out. Because if it fell out, it couldn't be donated. I figured I may as well get it cut so it could help someone else.

September 29

I've heard a phrase repeated over and over throughout this trial: "You have such a good attitude!"

"Me?" I ask. I've never had people tell me that. Sure,

I've had lots of people tell me I'm funny. But I've *never* had anyone tell me I have a good attitude. It makes me feel dirty. It's against my nature. I just use humor and sarcasm as a self-defense mechanism. It's something I've done since childhood. Humor has been a great weapon. It has also been great ally.

It also didn't hurt being a hypochondriac. Now, I wouldn't recommend anyone be like me. I don't want the competition! But, if you can laugh you'll be better off. I promise! I know it's serious. I know it's not funny. But you don't have to be miserable. That's not good for you or your health. When people would ask me how I was, I would say great! Don't revel in your misery. Save that for the new friends you make in chemo and radiation. You'll find it comforting making fun of all the people *without* cancer – with them!

Just like I recommend listening to music in radiation, you need to watch comedies on Netflix in chemo. There were a lot of people in chemo. I was one of the few that were laughing. Oh, I *know* I annoyed people. Look, it's not fun, and I understand that. But you may as well do something to get your mind off the fact there are needles in your arm and poison dripping into your veins!

I went to my friend, Joy, and she cut a foot of my hair off. It felt weird. I hadn't had short hair since fourth grade! I figured if it's cut off at least it can be made into a wig. If it falls out it'll be of no use to anyone.

September 30

I broke down on the radiation machine today. I don't know why. Apparently I just needed to cry. I started to panic. Now, keep in mind, I'm five feet off the ground when the machine is on. I was tapping my hands and moving. The technicians knew something was wrong. One of them came on the microphone. "Are you okay in there?"

"No!" I said.

"Hold tight, we will be right in," she said.

They both came in and I just lost it. I can't even write this now without crying. Before I had cancer, in the fifteen years my husband and I have been together, he'd only seen me cry twice. I am not a crier! They assured me that this happens to all their patients. I don't know why. I just started thinking about being halfway through. It didn't help that someone had ended their treatments and rang a bell to let everyone know it was their last time. I asked if I could give the techs a hug. ME! Oh God, on top of having cancer, *now I'm turning into a hugger!*

It's Wednesday so I have to meet with my physician's assistant. Everything is routine. He asks me the same questions as every other week: How are you feeling? Are you experiencing any burning? Are you in pain? Is your skin getting darker in the area being radiated? Are you feeling fatigued? Blah, blah, blah. The answers to those were no. I was still having minor nausea but not enough to complain about.

"Have you inserted anything in to your vagina?" he asked seriously.

Then, like all mature ladies my age, I started giggling and then got serious and asked, *"Such as…?"*

He went on to explain that radiation causes the tissue to atrophy and if I wasn't having regular sex that it would be too painful to have it all. And if that happened, he said they'd have to use a "device" to stretch me out. I wish I could show you the face I made at that comment.

"What kind of 'device' are you talking about?" I ask, not really wanting to know the answer.

He danced around the answer so much you would've thought he was walking on hot sand.

"It's uh…essentially, it's…" I raised my eyebrows and leaned in, waiting for the answer. "*A plastic penis*," he said. This incited more laughing from me.

"Would you be opposed to me using a *real* penis for this?" I asked.

"It might hurt," he said.

"I'll take my chances," I said. Then he wrote the name of a good lubricant down. He told me to get on top so I could control the situation. He reminded me to be gentle. That's funny. I'm having sex in the exact place I have cancer – *while* I'm still being treated for it. Yeah, I'll *consider* being gentle. Ha!

See, *now* I feel like I'm getting to know you!

Everything was fine. But I have to tell you, I had a huge mental block when it came to sex. It's hard not to think about cancer especially when it's below the equator.

We also talked about my weight gain – which did not make me laugh. Unlike most chemo patients, I didn't lose my appetite. Patients sometimes complain of a metallic taste in their mouths. Not me! Everything tasted great. As a result I was consistently going up in weight at every check-up. He assured me that they didn't want me losing weight during the treatment anyway. Ha! Fat chance of that happening…apparently.

Breast Cancer is the Prom Queen of All Cancers

Did you know that October is also Liver Cancer Awareness month? I bet you didn't. Breast Cancer, while be it serious…leaves the rest of us cancer patients wondering why is *she* the favorite? All cancers are ugly and deadly. Why does she get all of the attention? By the way, men are being diagnosed with breast cancer more than ever. I'm sure they *love* the pink ribbon.

Speaking of breasts, boys are getting too much soy in their diets. Too much soy leads to other problems. Such as early puberty, hormonal imbalances, mood swings, and man boobs. I hope you're not thinking, "Man boobs?

Good, that's one less present I'll have to buy little Billy for his birthday." Seriously, you have to realize that a poor diet contributes to health problems. Can the cure for cancer be in our diet? I don't know, but I have to believe that poor diet and exercise have to be a contributing factor of some forms of cancer.

Back to "the cure." Like me, I'm sure you have handed your money over to buy a t-shirt or pen to support "the cure." What you may not have known, and I only found out because of my own cancer education, is that most breast cancer "charities" are *for profit*. This means there's no accountability for how they spend your money. Many "charities" don't have much accountability either. If you want to support a legitimate cancer charity, please speak with someone at a cancer center. They would be happy to point you in the direction of a charity with low-overhead who is using money to fund research to actually find a cure. You can go to these sites: www.charitynavigator.org, www.charitywatch.org, or www.nasconet.org to research charities.

I team with two local charities who are honest non-profits that benefit breast cancer patients and survivors.

They are www.stretchitoutenterprise.org and www.teampinkswfl.org. I like to promote them and their hard work to make up for calling them prom queens!

The Number One Deadliest Cancer in America is…lung cancer. I know. I was surprised too. But, all cancer is deadly at some point. So, shouldn't we focus on eradicating *all* types of cancer?

However, the number one killing cancer for women in third-world countries is…my cancer. Where's all the love for cervical cancer? I want the NFL to wear teal and white. They only wear pink. That's not fair! It doesn't make sense, does it?

October 1

I decided I was going to make a list of all the things I wanted to do. This is important! Make plans. You will want something to look forward to. It will give you something to day dream about in chemo and radiation. Unfortunately, as I was writing this list, I noticed eyelashes were falling on the paper I was writing on. You know how you're supposed to make a wish on an eyelash? I wished they'd stop falling out. I hate cancer. I wouldn't wish it on anyone.

There will be days that you second-guess your treatment options. But remember this, cancer won't wait for your decision on how to treat it. It will continue to grow as you are weighing your options. My advice is discuss it with professionals and anyone you know that has been through cancer. One of the guys who works in radiation told me his wife's cancer story. If people that work in the cancer field didn't believe in these treatments, they wouldn't work there.

October 5

The nurses in chemo couldn't get a blood return. That's when they put the needle in and blood comes back out a tube. It's so they make sure the chemo is going directly into your blood stream, otherwise you could have permanent joint damage. They are putting arsenic in you! They poked me five times. They had to call the doctor and he said I had to come back the next day. I heard the word "port" several times, and I panicked. I only had two more treatments. I do not want a port put in! If you don't know what that is, you don't want to. If you have to have a port put in, it's not a big deal. Forget I even mentioned it. Eek.

When we got home, my husband in all his sensitivity, asked me if I'd like to get poked a sixth time. And people say romance is dead. Fools!

My neighbor came over with dinner. This was so nice because it was unexpected. That reminds me, don't forget to write thank you cards to people who do things for you during your time of need. Cancer is no excuse for bad manners!

October 6

I went back to chemo today, but I did my homework first. I researched on the internet about chemo patients not being able to have treatment because of their veins disappearing. I did not want a port so I was going to be a good little patient and figure out how I could make them appear. There was a little list someone was kind enough to put on the internet. You can do push-ups (I did standing ones against the wall in the elevator on the way up), wear warm clothes (if you're cold, your veins constrict), stay hydrated (I drank at least 400 ml of water before my treatment).

And it worked! As soon as the nurses saw me sit down, the ones that couldn't get a vein the previous day, came over and saw them sticking out. I told them I did push-ups in the elevator. They immediately stuck a needle in and got a blood return. Yay!

October 7

My physician's assistant and I discuss how I am. He asks about what we discussed last week. And then asks how the nausea is. I tell him I am eating a lot of crackers and toast when I'm nauseous. He notes I must be very nauseous. I ask him about a little black spot which has shown up on my right breast. He advises me to go to a dermatologist and have it looked at and then, if it's cancer, my oncologist will take care of it. Now that I have had cancer, I have to be really proactive when it comes to future potential problems. I inform him that I have a friend that is a dermatological cancer surgeon. Granted, I am not in the habit of showing my friends my breasts but there is a first time for everything.

October 9

I get on the elevator with a gentleman. He pressed the floor for chemo. I noticed it and said, "Gross. I don't want to go to that floor. Everyone on that floor has cancer."

"Where you going then?" he asked as he leaned in to press a button for me.

"The same floor. I have cancer, too," I said with a smirk. He just laughed at me.

Actually, I *was* happy about it. It was the last time I was getting my chemo blood draw. Yay!

October 12

My last chemo! My blood pressure was high all morning. And my heart rate was high, too. Last week anxiety. Again, it's normal to be stressed out. The girls in chemo were so funny. They all signed a certificate of completion for me. I will miss them. I'm also glad I won't have to see them again. But, they were a fun group of people. It takes a special person to work with cancer patients.

October 13

When I walked into the cancer building, the smell of fish slapped me in the face. While normally I appreciate the fact that the deli downstairs has fresh food, when you are already nauseous from chemo you don't want to smell that!

October 15

It was a surprisingly emotional day at radiation. When you have your final session they let you ring a bell and the staff claps and give you hugs. Wow. I really lost it. I was a mess when I walked out of that building. I didn't have to see my physician's assistant that day. I did get an appointment with my radiation doctor for the next month. I was hesitant to declare myself cancer-free again! I wrap up my cancer treatment almost fifteen pounds heavier than when I started. So much for *losing* weight on chemo.

When your treatment is done it is a good time to go to the vitamin store and buy a pharmaceutical grade probiotic for your stomach. In the process of killing cancer, the innocent and good bacteria in your stomach has been killed as well! You have to put those little suckers back!

You are also going to need to clean out your fridge and pantry. Depending on how long your treatments were, you may have a lot of expired food in your home. I did!

October 30

I finally call about the spot on my breast. I get an appointment for the next week.

November 3

I go see my skin doctor in Port Charlotte. If I have skin

cancer now, *God help me*, he can take care of it. But more importantly, he's funny. And if I'm going to get more bad news I'd rather get it from someone I know and who has my sense of humor. I tell him the harrowing tale of my cancer experience prompting all of the "oohs" and "ahs" a good storyteller expects at their appropriate times. I told him how they thought they'd be able to remove it with surgery alone and then when the pathology report came back I had to have chemo and radiation because it had spread. He said he was sorry I had to go through all that and I said it was all right. My experience would make a better book now. He just laughed and said only I would think that's okay and worth it for the book!

While he's examining me, he comments on how small it is (the spot, not my breast) and then adds that he's surprised that I could see something so small turning black. I told him that I looked at it under a jeweler's loupe – which made him laugh. I told him I even came up with a new slogan for them, "Jeweler's Loupes, Not Just for Diamonds." He told me almost instantly that even if it was cancer, which he didn't believe it was, it was so small that it would be nothing. He told me not to lose sleep over it.

November 7

I was talking with a friend and fellow cancer survivor, whom I met at radiation. She asked me about the progress of this book. I said, "I need to hurry and finish because I just got my first speaking engagement in January to speak about being a cancer survivor."

"Ugh, I hate that term 'cancer survivor.' Don't you hate being called that?" she asked.

"Not at all. You know what they'd call me if they didn't call me that?" I said.

"No. What?" she inquired.

"Dead!" I said with a laugh.

"Well, I'm not telling anyone I'm a cancer survivor," she said.

"That's your business and I won't tell anyone, but there will come a time where you will have to tell someone. God allowed you to go through this so you could help someone else," I said.

November 10

My skin doctor's office called and said the biopsy came back clear. Thank God. I really can't take any more bad news.

November 11

I got the all clear from my radiation oncologist. He said I should just go back to living life like normal. Maybe go on an adventure. My husband asked where I wanted to go for dinner to celebrate and I said, "Five Guys!" I know, I'm a cheap date. After I ate a big cheeseburger and about fifty French fries, we contemplated what we would do next. I asked him to take my picture at Five Guys, which I posted to Facebook. I told him I should go see grandpa but I didn't want to. So, *I didn't*. There was always tomorrow.

I guess you know what I'm going to tell you next. It's almost predictable. Grandpa died later that night. And you're probably thinking what everyone else said to me. He wouldn't have even known whether I showed up or not. But, *I* knew! No one is promised tomorrow. I should know that more than anyone. I was so sorry I didn't make the time to say goodbye. I hadn't seen him since his birthday and now I was even fatter. He really wouldn't have recognized me this time.

Things to keep in mind for friends and families of cancer patients:

- Cancer is not the only thing we want to talk about.
- We are not "cancer victims." I hate that term. We are regular people who are embroiled in a battle for our lives.
- We need to laugh. Please bring us funny movies and stories when you come to visit.
- Don't dump your problems on us. Hey, we have cancer. That's enough to deal with.
- Join a support group for cancer caregivers so can unburden yourself without burdening us!
- Bring us a meal or help us with laundry. We are tired and cranky but we have a good reason!
- Don't post or forward pics of people in chemo on Facebook and say "like" the picture if you care, or

ignore if you're heartless. Seriously? I got these all the time while *I* was in chemo. I may have "accidently" unfriended some people who posted this kind of crap.

- Don't pity us. We will outlive many of you!

As I put up the Christmas tree, Wi-Fi ran under it and lay down and napped right on Samson's old spot on the satin tree skirt. And for the few hours a day she was awake, she made sure she swatted at all of the ornaments that Samson had batted around for the previous Christmases. Looking at her, I'm reminded of Samson and realize if he hadn't been so thirsty I wouldn't have noticed my own body giving me a clue that something was wrong. Maybe he died so I wouldn't.

Can you imagine someone sacrificing themselves for you? It's not the first time it's happened in history. And it may have not been the reason Samson died. But in my heart I will always believe his life was given for mine.

As we celebrated Thanksgiving, there was noticeably an empty chair at the dinner table. I missed grandpa's hearty laugh when I said something inappropriate. But, he was ninety and had a long life. And, he was loved.

I guess I was depressed about the year because after our Thanksgiving meal, I ate a half of a pecan pie, while standing alone in the kitchen when everyone else was distracted by football. But in my defense, I love pecan pie. I was no longer depressed about cancer. I was depressed I still hadn't regained the pee warning signal. I doubted it would ever return now.

By the time Christmas rolled around, I had gained five more pounds. The cancer may be gone but now I will have to work hard to lose the weight I gained through the year.

Instead of remembering all I lost this year, I think about what I still have left. Some of the people I met in chemo and radiation weren't as lucky as I was. So, as 2015 draws to a close, I decided not to look back at it as the worst year of my life. Instead I will look back at 2015 as a year that could've been so much worse. And if by chance we should ever meet, go ahead…give me a hug!

ABOUT THE AUTHOR

Angelina is an award-winning humor writer of fiction novels. This is Angelina's first non-fiction book. She lives in Fort Myers and is working on other humor novels. Because life is too short to not be laughing.

Follow Angelina on Twitter

@lotteryheiress

Visit her website

www.thelotteryheiress.com

Visit her on Facebook

Facebook.com/angelinaassanti

Email her

angassanti@gmail.com

Made in the USA
Columbia, SC
02 September 2017